YOUR KNOWLEDGE HAS VALUE

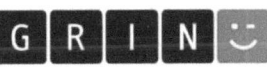

Risk of Subsequent Adjacent Fractures after Vertebral Augmentation in the Treatment for Osteoporotic Vertebral Compression Fractures

José Manuel Ortega Zufiría
Rosa María Benítez Clemente
Aida Yuste Sánchez

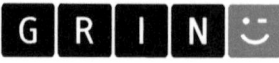

Bibliographic information published by the German National Library:

The German National Library lists this publication in the National Bibliography; detailed bibliographic data are available on the Internet at http://dnb.dnb.de.

ISBN: 9783346289063
This book is also available as an ebook.

© GRIN Publishing GmbH
Nymphenburger Straße 86
80636 München

Print and binding: Books on Demand GmbH, Norderstedt, Germany
Printed on acid-free paper from responsible sources.

The present work has been carefully prepared. Nevertheless, authors and publishers do not incur liability for the correctness of information, notes, links and advice as well as any printing errors.

GRIN web shop: https://www.grin.com/document/948546

Risk of Subsequent Adjacent Fractures after Vertebral Augmentation in the Treatment for Osteoporotic Vertebral Compression Fractures: a Systematic Review and Meta-Analysis.

José Manuel Ortega Zufiría
Rosa María Benítez Clemente
Aida Yuste Sánchez

INDEX	

ABSTRACT:

Objectives:

The aim of this study was to investigate whether percutaneous vertebral augmentation (PVA) was associated with clinical and radiological subsequent adjacent fractures.

Patients and Methods:

A systematic review and meta-analysis was performed searching on PubMed, EMBASE, Cochrane library, Google Scholar, web of science and ClinicalTrial.gov from the establishment of the database to January 2020. Eligible studies assessing the subsequent adjacent fractures after PVA compared with conservative treatment (CT) were incorporated. The pooled risk ratio (RR) with its 95% confidence intervals (95% CI) was used. Heterogeneity, sensitivity and publication bias analyses were performed.

Results:

24 studies were considered eligible and were included finally. 20/421 patients (4.75%) had clinical subsequent adjacent fractures from PVA group, and 25/359 patients (6.96%) had from CT group, and 46/440 patients (10.45%) from PVA group and 36/444 patients (8.10%) from CT group had radiological subsequent adjacent fractures. There both had no significant difference between two groups (RR=0.67, 95%CI: [0.38, 1.19], P = 0.17)/ (RR=1.13, 95%CI: [0.75, 1.70], P = 0.576). However, in fractured vertebrae, number in PVA group was more than that in CT group (RR=1.41, 95%CI: [1.03, 1.93], P = 0.03).

Conclusion:

Collectively, currently available literature provides data showed PVA did not increase the incidence for subsequent adjacent fractures, no matter it was clinical or radiological fracture. But PVA may increase the number of fractured vertebrae.

Abbreviations:

OVCF: osteoporotic vertebral compression fracture

PVA: percutaneous vertebral augmentation

PVP: percutaneous vertebroplasty

PKP: percutaneous kyphoplasty

CT: conservative treatment

RCT: randomized controlled trial

RR: risk ratio

CI: confidence interval

1 INTRODUCTION:

As one of the most common complications of osteoporosis, osteoporotic vertebral compression fractures (OVCFs) often results in back pain, spinal deformity, functional disability, and even death. So it has become one of the serious diseases threatening the health of elderly patients and increased the economic burden of society [1,2,5,7].

As a minimally invasive therapy for OVCFs, percutaneous vertebral augmentation (PVA) has shown promising and encouraging outcomes compared with conservative treatment (CT) [2, 3,4,6].

Moreover, according to different feature of fracture, PVA can choose percutaneous vertebroplasty (PVP), percutaneous kyphoplasty (PKP) or other operation methods. However, PVA can also lead to serious complications, the most serious of which is subsequent fracture, so the efficacy and safety of PVA are still in dispute [5,8,9,10]. The subsequent fractures can occur at adjacent, non-adjacent or even previously treated vertebral levels.

However, there were few meta-analyses [1,12,13,14,15,36] only to probe subsequent adjacent fractures, and RCTs as much as possible were not included in those reviews.

Furthermore, none of these studies distinguished clinical and radiological fracture, as well as the number of fractured patients and fractured vertebrae for analysis (16,17,18,19). The purpose of this study is to explore the characteristics of subsequent adjacent fracture after PVA, so as to provide evidence for the treatment strategy of OVCF (20,21, 28, 35).

2   MATERIAL AND METHODS:

Search strategy and study selection:

Two independent reviewers respectively conducted rough and accurate computerized retrieval in online databases, including PubMed, EMBASE, Cochrane library, Google Scholar, web of science and ClinicalTrial.gov, from the establishment of the database to January 2020.

We also searched references to selected literatures to avoid missing any additional research.

There are no language restrictions when searching (Fig. 1).

Rough search strategy: (vertebroplasty OR kyphoplasty OR vertebral augmentation) AND (conservative treatment) AND ((new fracture) OR (secondary fracture) OR (subsequent fracture) OR (adjacent fracture)).

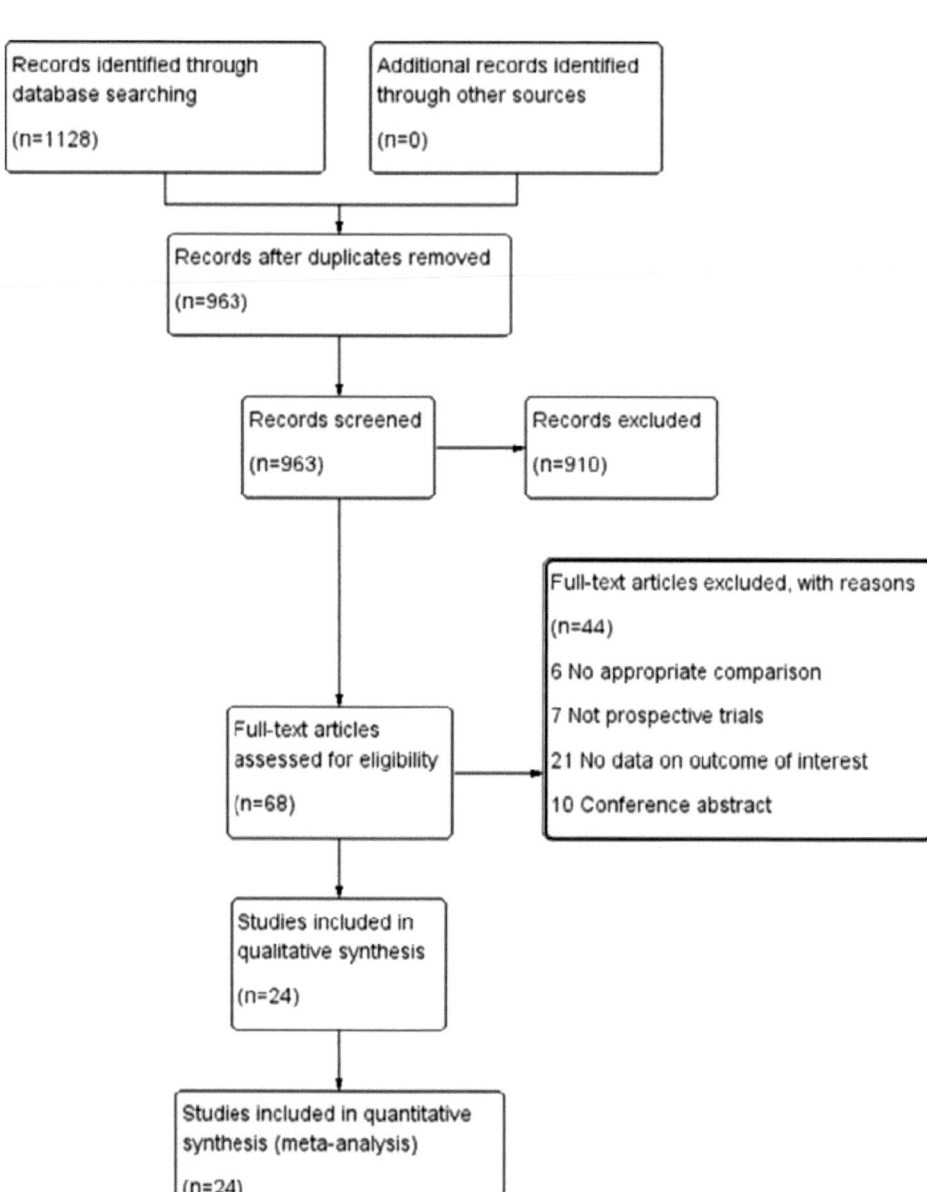

Figure 1.

Inclusion criteria:

Participants:

Only adult patients (age ≥ 50 years old) diagnosed with OVCF by clinical and imaging examination were included.

Intervention and control:

PVA (PVP/PKP) was performed in the experimental group and CT (including sham operation) was performed in the control group.

Outcomes:

The incidence of subsequent adjacent vertebral fractures. Study type: Prospective cohort study, Non-RCT, and RCT.

Study selection and data extraction:

Endnote X9 software was used to check, sort and summarize the literatures; then each study was carefully read and selected by two independent reviewers by double-blind method. Any disagreement was resolved by discussion or by consulting a third reviewer. The number of clinical and radiological subsequent adjacent fracture were separately extracted and classified.

If subsequent adjacent fracture did not have clear definition in the article, we deal with it as radiological fracture, because most fractures need imaging to be diagnosed. If patient had subsequent adjacent vertebral fractures equal to or more than two levels at once time, we just counted once for incidence.

Risk of bias assessment and quality evaluation:

Two independent reviewers applied the risk of bias tool to appraise all the included literatures according to the Cochrane Handbook for Systematic Reviews of Interventions (version 5.1.0), respectively. The methodological quality was assessed according to the

8

Cochrane Collaboration's domain-based evaluation framework [12, 13]. The main domains were assessed in the following sequence: (1) selection bias (randomized sequence generation and allocation concealment), (2) performance bias (blinding of participants and personnel), (3) detection bias (blinding of outcome assessment), (4) attrition bias (incomplete outcome data, e.g., due to dropouts), (5) reporting bias (selective reporting), and (6) other sources of bias. The score for each bias domain and the final score for the risk of systematic bias were graded as representing low, high, or unclear risk.

According to the Jadad scale [14], the quality of RCTs was evaluated, including the following four aspects: (1) Generation of random sequence; (2) Allocation concealment; (3) Implementation of blind method; (4) Description of case follow-up. "1-3" was considered as low quality, and "4-7" was considered as high quality.

Statistical analysis:

To compare the differences from incidence for subsequent adjacent fractures after PVA, dichotomous data were calculated by risk ratio (RR) and its 95% confidence interval (95%CI). Heterogeneity was tested using the chi-squared statistic and the I2 statistic. If the $P < 0.1$, we defined the chi-squared statistic as statistically significant.

The I2 statistic was used to assess the variation across the included trails as the following standard: I2 < 25% means that heterogeneity is low; I2: 25-50% shows moderate heterogeneity; I2 > 50% demonstrates high heterogeneity. If I2 > 50%, a random-effect model would be adopted; otherwise, a fixed-effect model would be used [15].

Sensitivity analyses were conducted to investigate the impacts of each individual study by deleting them in turn on the overall meta-analysis results. Publication bias was detected using the method of Begg's and Egger's test. The statistical analysis was performed by Review Manager 5.3 and Stata 15.0.

9

3   RESULTS:

Description of studies:

From the PRISMA Flow Diagram, the search and selection process of related literatures in this study were described. A total of 1128 literatures were retrieved, and 68 literatures were evaluated according to the inclusion criteria. Finally, 14 serial studies (total 24 literatures, including 5 serial non-RCTs [16-23] and 9 serial RCTs [24-38]) were selected.

Risk of bias and quality evaluation of included studies:

Because cement is opaque in imaging, it is difficult to blind patients, surgeons and observers, so only two of the serial studies (Control group had sham operation) were blinded to the patients. Six serial studies reported an adequate blinding for outcomes assessors. From the Jadad scale, eight serial studies [16, 20, 21, 24-35, 37, 38,41,43] were considered as high quality, and the others were considered as low quality.

Meta-analysis results:

The incidence of clinical subsequent adjacent fractures after PVA:

A total of 20/421 patients (4.75%) had clinical subsequent adjacent fractures from PVA group, and 25/359 patients (6.96%) had from CT group. There showed no significant difference between two groups (RR=0.67, 95%CI: [0.38, 1.19], P = 0.17. M-H. Fixed-effect model, I2= 31%).

The incidence of radiological subsequent adjacent fractures after PVA:

As far as radiological subsequent adjacent fractures were concerned, the results showed that 46/440 patients (10.45%) from PVA group and 36/444 patients (8.10%) from CT group had this complication form. There always had no significant difference between two groups (RR=1.13, 95%CI: [0.75, 1.70], P = 0.576. M-H. Fixed-effect model, I2= 0%).

The number of subsequent adjacent fractures for vertebrae after PVA:

In number of fractured vertebrae, 69/126 vertebral bodies (54.76%) had subsequent adjacent fractures from PVA group and 40/105 vertebral bodies (38.10%) had from CT group. There showed a significant difference between two groups (RR=1.41, 95%CI: [1.03, 1.93], P =
0.03. M-H. Fixed-effect model, I2= 0%).

Sensitivity and publication bias analysis:

Sensitivity analyses were conducted due to the discrepancy between studies. Each study was removed in turn to test whether the removed study would influence the overall effects. No specific trials could be determined as the main source of heterogeneity.

From the results of publication bias, the results of Begg's test (clinical fractures: P= 0.707> 0.05/ radiological fractures: P= 0.806> 0.05/ fractures for vertebrae: P=0.086> 0.05) and Egger's test (clinical fractures: P= 0.599> 0.05/ radiological fractures: P= 0.659> 0.05/ fractures for vertebrae: P= 0.061> 0.05) did not indicate the existence of publication bias.

4   DISCUSSIONS:

With the advantage of pain relief rapidly, PVA, as a minimally invasive technique, has become the most popular treatment for OVCFs. However, PVA also has some complications and risks, such as cement leakage and subsequent fractures.

The incidence of cement leakage is high, but most of them are asymptomatic, so it is generally believed that the cement leakage is a phenomenon rather than a complication. But subsequent fracture is different.

Once it happens, it will seriously influence the effect of PVA. About the reason, no convincing conclusion has been obtained from current studies, including biomechanical research, finite element analysis and clinical studies [21,23,27,33,35,36,39-43]. Many

11

meta-analyses [6, 8-11,37-41,43,46,47] have shown that subsequent fracture is related to the natural progression of osteoporosis, not due to the PVA with cement. However, only one [7] has detailed the influence on subsequent adjacent vertebral fractures after PVA.

The most remarkable differences from the previous meta-analysis were that clinical and radiological subsequent adjacent fracture, as well as the number of fractured cases and fractured vertebrae were analyzed separately. Because OVCFs were mostly caused by minor trauma, and some elderly patients were not sensitive to pain. If regular imaging examinations were not taken, misdiagnosis was inevitable.

The clinical subsequent fractures and radiological ones are separately analyzed in this study, which was more persuasive. Moreover, if patient had equal to or more than two fractured levels at once time, it only showed the more number of subsequent adjacent vertebral fractures, not the increasing frequency, so we just counted once for incidence.

This study showed that no significant differences were in the incidence of subsequent adjacent fractures between PVA and CT, regardless of fracture type, which came to conclusion that PVA was a safe and feasible treatment for OVCF, and would not increase the risk of secondary adjacent fracture (21,23,46,47). However, the number of vertebrae fractured in PVA group was more than that in CT group, which meant the severity was worse.

Firstly, although the clinical characteristics at baseline in those studies were similar, (Except for Klazen's study, the number of OVCFs at baseline was statistically significant (2.4±1.9 vs 2.1±1.5)) the number of OVCFs and severity of fracture at baseline in PVA group were worse than that in CT group.

Secondly, because of more vertebral body fractures, the phenomenon of "sandwich type" after PVA would increase. As a special type of OVCF, it may lead to subsequent adjacent fractures more easily.

Thirdly, because rapidly relieve pain, the patients after PVA can make exercise early, so trauma without awareness of protection and short-term treatment of anti-osteoporosis would increase risk.

In addition, this study had incorporated some non-RCTs. As an adverse effect, subsequent fractures were objective outcomes during the follow-up and would not be obviously affected by randomization and blinding method, which may not influence the reliability too much. This can increased the sample size and made it more convincing.

In sensitivity analysis, no apparent deviation was observed in all trials included, indicating that no specific trial influenced the overall effects. From the results of Begg's and Egger's test, potential publication bias was not found. It showed RCTs of poor quality and non-RCTs would still provide relatively accurate data for subsequent fractures as an objective outcome from another aspect.

Limitation:

There also had some limitations in our study. Firstly, subgroup analysis was not done by different operation methods (PVP/PKP), follow-up time. Because this review compared clinical fracture and radiological one separately, so there were few eligible literatures for subgroup analysis. For another, previous studies had clearly shown the factors above that has no effect on subsequent fractures. Secondly, most studies mainly focused on pain relief and functional recovery, so other influence factors for subsequent fractures are not considered, such as age, sex, low body mass index, the fracture age, cement leakage, bilateral or unilateral, multiple levels treated, the volume of cement, anti-osteoporosis treatment and low bone mineral density [44-47]. Therefore, further RCTs of high quality, large sample size, long term follow-up between PVA and CT were demanded to offer more invaluable and convincing conclusion.

5. CONCLUSION:

In conclusion, PVA may not increase the incidence for subsequent adjacent fractures, no matter it was clinical or radiological fracture. It might be related to the natural process of osteoporosis, as there are spinal zones where risk is considered to be increased across several levels simultaneously. But PVA may increase the number of fractured vertebrae.

Ethics approval and consent to participate:

The study was approved by the Institutional Review Board. All procedures performed in studies involving human participants were in accordance with the ethical standards of the institutional and/or national research committee and with the 1964 Helsinki declaration and its later amendments or comparable ethical standards.

REFERENCES:

1. Lyritis GP. The history of the walls of the Acropolis of Athens and the natural history of secondary fracture healing process. J Musculoskelet Neuronal Interact 2000;1:1-3.
2. Mattie R, Laimi K, Yu S, Saltychev M. Comparing Percutaneous Vertebroplasty and Conservative Therapy for Treating Osteoporotic Compression Fractures in the Thoracic and Lumbar Spine: A Systematic Review and Meta-Analysis. J BONE JOINT SURG AM 2016;98:1041-1051.
3. Stevenson M, Gomersall T, Lloyd JM, Rawdin A, Hernandez M, Dias S, Wilson D, Rees A. Percutaneous vertebroplasty and percutaneous balloon kyphoplasty for the treatment of osteoporotic vertebral fractures: a systematic review and cost-effectiveness analysis. Health Technol Assess 2014;18:1-290.
4. Fribourg D, Tang C, Sra P, Delamarter R, Bae H. Incidence of subsequent vertebral fracture after kyphoplasty. Spine (Phila Pa 1976) 2004;29:2270-2276, 2277.
5. Lee BG, Choi JH, Kim DY, Choi WR, Lee SG, Kang CN. Risk factors for newly developed osteoporotic vertebral compression fractures following treatment for osteoporotic vertebral compression fractures. SPINE J 2019;19:301-305.
6. Bouza C, Lopez-Cuadrado T, Almendro N, Amate JM. Safety of balloon kyphoplasty in the treatment of osteoporotic vertebral compression fractures in Europe: a meta-analysis of randomized controlled trials. EUR SPINE J 2015;24:715-723.
7. Fan B, Wei Z, Zhou X, Lin W, Ren Y, Li A, Shi G, Hao Y, Liu S, Zhou H, Feng S. Does vertebral augmentation lead to an increasing incidence of adjacent vertebral failure? A systematic review and meta-analysis. INT J SURG 2016;36:369-376.

8.   Li HM, Zhang RJ, Gao H, Jia CY, Zhang JX, Dong FL, Shen CL. New vertebral fractures after osteoporotic vertebral compression fracture between balloon kyphoplasty and nonsurgical treatment PRISMA. Medicine (Baltimore) 2018;97:e12666.

9.   Marcia S, Muto M, Hirsch JA, Chandra RV, Carter N, Crivelli P, Piras E, Saba L. What is the role of vertebral augmentation for osteoporotic fractures? A review of the recent literature. NEURORADIOLOGY 2018;60:777-783.

10.   Zhu RS, Kan SL, Ning GZ, Chen LX, Cao ZG, Jiang ZH, Zhang XL, Hu W. Which is the best treatment of osteoporotic vertebral compression fractures: balloon kyphoplasty, percutaneous vertebroplasty, or non-surgical treatment? A Bayesian network meta-analysis. Osteoporos Int 2019;30:287-298.

11.   Zuo XH, Zhu XP, Bao HG, Xu CJ, Chen H, Gao XZ, Zhang QX. Network meta-analysis of percutaneous vertebroplasty, percutaneous kyphoplasty, nerve block, and conservative treatment for nonsurgery options of acute/subacute and chronic osteoporotic vertebral compression fractures (OVCFs) in short-term and long-term effects. Medicine (Baltimore) 2018;97:e11544.

12.   Cumpston M, Li T, Page MJ, Chandler J, Welch VA, Higgins JP, Thomas J. Updated guidance for trusted systematic reviews: a new edition of the Cochrane Handbook for Systematic Reviews of Interventions. Cochrane Database Syst Rev 2019;10:D142.

13.   Saltychev M, Mikkelsson M, Laimi K. Medication of inclusion body myositis: a systematic review. ACTA NEUROL SCAND 2016;133:97-102.

14.   Jadad AR, Moore RA, Carroll D, Jenkinson C, Reynolds DJ, Gavaghan DJ, McQuay HJ. Assessing the quality of reports of randomized clinical trials: is blinding necessary? Control Clin Trials 1996;17:1-12.

15.   Higgins JP, Thompson SG, Deeks JJ, Altman DG. Measuring inconsistency in meta-analyses. BMJ 2003;327:557-560.

16.   Du JP, Fan Y, Liu JJ, Zhang JN, Huang YS, Zhang J, Hao DJ. The analysis of MSTMOVCF (Multi-segment thoracolumbar mild osteoporotic fractures surgery or conservative treatment) based on ASTLOF (the assessment system of thoracolumbar osteoporotic fracture). Sci Rep 2018;8:8185.

17.   Diamond TH, Bryant C, Browne L, Clark WA. Clinical outcomes after acute osteoporotic vertebral fractures: a 2-year non-randomised trial comparing percutaneous vertebroplasty with conservative therapy. Med J Aust 2006;184:113-117.

18. Diamond TH, Champion B, Clark WA. Management of acute osteoporotic vertebral fractures: a nonrandomized trial comparing percutaneous vertebroplasty with conservative therapy. AM J MED 2003;114:257-265.

19. Grafe IA, Da FK, Hillmeier J, Meeder PJ, Libicher M, Noldge G, Bardenheuer H, Pyerin W, Basler L, Weiss C, Taylor RS, Nawroth P, Kasperk C. Reduction of pain and fracture incidence after kyphoplasty: 1-year outcomes of a prospective controlled trial of patients with primary osteoporosis. Osteoporos Int 2005;16:2005-2012.

20. Kasperk C, Grafe IA, Schmitt S, Noldge G, Weiss C, Da FK, Hillmeier J, Libicher M, Sommer U, Rudofsky G, Meeder PJ, Nawroth P. Three-year outcomes after kyphoplasty in patients with osteoporosis with painful vertebral fractures. J VASC INTERV RADIOL 2010;21:701-709.

21. Kasperk C, Hillmeier J, Noldge G, Grafe IA, Dafonseca K, Raupp D, Bardenheuer H, Libicher M, Liegibel UM, Sommer U, Hilscher U, Pyerin W, Vetter M, Meinzer HP, Meeder PJ, Taylor RS, Nawroth P. Treatment of painful vertebral fractures by kyphoplasty in patients with primary osteoporosis: a prospective nonrandomized controlled study. J BONE MINER RES 2005;20:604-612.

22. Movrin I. Adjacent level fracture after osteoporotic vertebral compression fracture: a nonrandomized prospective study comparing balloon kyphoplasty with conservative therapy. WIEN KLIN WOCHENSCHR 2012;124:304-311.

23. Wang HK, Lu K, Liang CL, Weng HC, Wang KW, Tsai YD, Hsieh CH, Liliang PC. Comparing clinical outcomes following percutaneous vertebroplasty with conservative therapy for acute osteoporotic vertebral compression fractures. PAIN MED 2010;11:1659-1665.

24. Blasco J, Martinez-Ferrer A, Macho J, San RL, Pomes J, Carrasco J, Monegal A, Guanabens N, Peris P. Effect of vertebroplasty on pain relief, quality of life, and the incidence of new vertebral fractures: a 12-month randomized follow-up, controlled trial. J BONE MINER RES 2012;27:1159-1166.

25. Boonen S, Van Meirhaeghe J, Bastian L, Cummings SR, Ranstam J, Tillman JB, Eastell R, Talmadge K, Wardlaw D. Balloon kyphoplasty for the treatment of acute vertebral compression fractures: 2-year results from a randomized trial. J BONE MINER RES 2011;26:1627-1637.

26. Buchbinder R, Osborne RH, Ebeling PR, Wark JD, Mitchell P, Wriedt C, Graves S, Staples MP, Murphy B. A randomized trial of vertebroplasty for painful osteoporotic vertebral fractures. N Engl J Med 2009;361:557-568.

27. Farrokhi MR, Alibai E, Maghami Z. Randomized controlled trial of percutaneous vertebroplasty versus optimal medical management for the relief of pain and disability in acute osteoporotic vertebral compression fractures. J Neurosurg Spine 2011;14:561-569.

28. Firanescu CE, de Vries J, Lodder P, Schoemaker MC, Smeets AJ, Donga E, Juttmann JR, Klazen C, Elgersma O, Jansen FH, van der Horst I, Blonk M, Venmans A, Lohle P. Percutaneous Vertebroplasty is no Risk Factor for New Vertebral Fractures and Protects Against Further Height Loss (VERTOS IV). Cardiovasc Intervent Radiol 2019;42:991-1000.

29. Firanescu CE, de Vries J, Lodder P, Venmans A, Schoemaker MC, Smeets AJ, Donga E, Juttmann JR, Klazen C, Elgersma O, Jansen FH, Tielbeek AV, Boukrab I, Schonenberg K, van Rooij W, Hirsch JA, Lohle P. Vertebroplasty versus sham procedure for painful acute osteoporotic vertebral compression fractures (VERTOS IV): randomised sham controlled clinical trial. BMJ 2018;361:k1551.

30. Kroon F, Staples M, Ebeling PR, Wark JD, Osborne RH, Mitchell PJ, Wriedt CH, Buchbinder R. Two-year results of a randomized placebo-controlled trial of vertebroplasty for acute osteoporotic vertebral fractures. J BONE MINER RES 2014;29:1346-1355.

31. Martinez-Ferrer A, Blasco J, Carrasco JL, Macho JM, Roman LS, Lopez A, Monegal A, Guanabens N, Peris P. Risk factors for the development of vertebral fractures after percutaneous vertebroplasty. J BONE MINER RES 2013;28:1821-1829.

32. Rousing R, Andersen MO, Jespersen SM, Thomsen K, Lauritsen J. Percutaneous vertebroplasty compared to conservative treatment in patients with painful acute or subacute osteoporotic vertebral fractures: three-months follow-up in a clinical randomized study. Spine (Phila Pa 1976) 2009;34:1349-1354.

33. Rousing R, Hansen KL, Andersen MO, Jespersen SM, Thomsen K, Lauritsen JM. Twelve-months follow-up in forty-nine patients with acute/semiacute osteoporotic vertebral fractures treated conservatively or with percutaneous vertebroplasty: a clinical randomized study. Spine (Phila Pa 1976) 2010;35:478-482.

34. Staples MP, Howe BM, Ringler MD, Mitchell P, Wriedt CH, Wark JD, Ebeling PR, Osborne RH, Kallmes DF, Buchbinder R. New vertebral fractures after vertebroplasty: 2-year results from a randomised controlled trial. ARCH OSTEOPOROS 2015;10:229.

17

35. Van Meirhaeghe J, Bastian L, Boonen S, Ranstam J, Tillman JB, Wardlaw D. A randomized trial of balloon kyphoplasty and nonsurgical management for treating acute vertebral compression fractures: vertebral body kyphosis correction and surgical parameters. Spine (Phila Pa 1976) 2013;38:971-983.

36. Voormolen MH, Mali WP, Lohle PN, Fransen H, Lampmann LE, van der Graaf Y, Juttmann JR, Jansssens X, Verhaar HJ. Percutaneous vertebroplasty compared with optimal pain medication treatment: short-term clinical outcome of patients with subacute or chronic painful osteoporotic vertebral compression fractures. The VERTOS study. AJNR Am J Neuroradiol 2007;28:555-560.

37. Wardlaw D, Cummings SR, Van Meirhaeghe J, Bastian L, Tillman JB, Ranstam J, Eastell R, Shabe P, Talmadge K, Boonen S. Efficacy and safety of balloon kyphoplasty compared with non-surgical care for vertebral compression fracture (FREE): a randomised controlled trial. LANCET 2009;373:1016-1024.

38. Yi X, Lu H, Tian F, Wang Y, Li C, Liu H, Liu X, Li H. Recompression in new levels after percutaneous vertebroplasty and kyphoplasty compared with conservative treatment. Arch Orthop Trauma Surg 2014;134:21-30.

39. Belkoff SM, Mathis JM, Jasper LE, Deramond H. An ex vivo biomechanical evaluation of a hydroxyapatite cement for use with vertebroplasty. Spine (Phila Pa 1976) 2001;26:1542-1546.

40. Fahim DK, Sun K, Tawackoli W, Mendel E, Rhines LD, Burton AW, Kim DH, Ehni BL, Liebschner MA. Premature adjacent vertebral fracture after vertebroplasty: a biomechanical study. NEUROSURGERY 2011;69:733-744.

41. Rohlmann A, Zander T, Bergmann G. Spinal loads after osteoporotic vertebral fractures treated by vertebroplasty or kyphoplasty. EUR SPINE J 2006;15:1255-1264.

42. Seel EH, Davies EM. A biomechanical comparison of kyphoplasty using a balloon bone tamp versus an expandable polymer bone tamp in a deer spine model. J Bone Joint Surg Br 2007;89:253-257.

43. Yang S, Liu Y, Yang H, Zou J. Risk factors and correlation of secondary adjacent vertebral compression fracture in percutaneous kyphoplasty. INT J SURG 2016;36:138-142.

44. Chen WJ, Kao YH, Yang SC, Yu SW, Tu YK, Chung KC. Impact of cement leakage into disks on the development of adjacent vertebral compression fractures. J SPINAL DISORD TECH 2010;23:35-39.

45.   Hiwatashi A, Westesson PL. Patients with osteoporosis on steroid medication tend to sustain subsequent fractures. AJNR Am J Neuroradiol 2007;28:1055-1057.

46.   Li YA, Lin CL, Chang MC, Liu CL, Chen TH, Lai SC. Subsequent vertebral fracture after vertebroplasty: incidence and analysis of risk factors. Spine (Phila Pa 1976) 2012;37:179-183.

47.   Sun G, Tang H, Li M, Liu X, Jin P, Li L. Analysis of risk factors of subsequent fractures after vertebroplasty. EUR SPINE J 2014;23:13

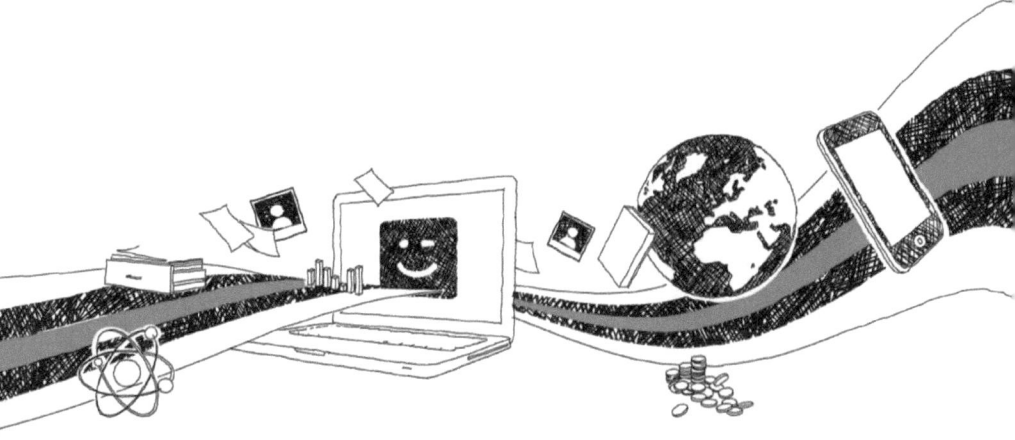
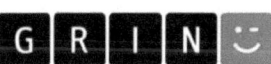

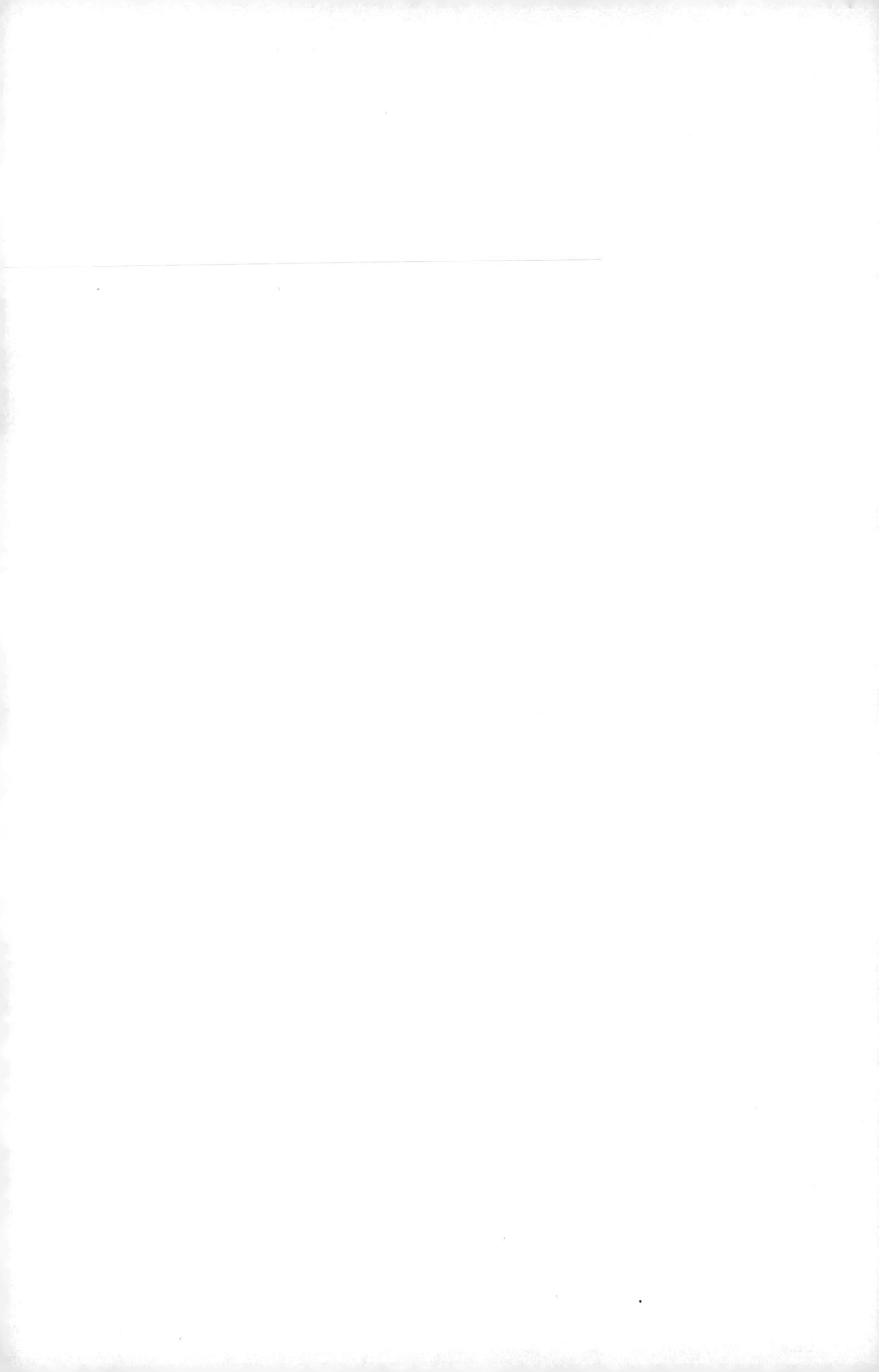